PARKINSON'S DISEASE DIET COOK BOOK

The Parkinson's Disease Diet: Ideal Food Selections for Managing Parkinson's Disease

LARRY HERMAN

Table of Contents

Introduction

Parkinson's Disease Is A Neurological Condition That Mostly Impacts The Ability To Move. It Is A Degenerative Disorder, Indicating That Symptoms Deteriorate As Time Passes. The Condition Is Named After James Parkinson, The British Physician Who Initially Documented Its Symptoms In 1817.

Notable Characteristics Of Parkinson's disease Include:

• Bradykinesia Is The Condition Characterized By A Reduced Speed Of Movement. People Diagnosed With Parkinson's Disease May Experience Challenges When Starting And Finishing Motions, Resulting In An

Overall Decrease In Their Ability To Move Rapidly.

- Resting Tremors Are Prevalent Symptoms That Typically Occur In The Hands, Fingers, Or Other Body Parts When The Body Is At Rest. Tremors May Diminish Or Cease When Intentional Movement Is Performed.

- **Rigidity:** The Presence Of Inflexibility In The Limbs And Joints Is Another Distinct Characteristic. Muscles Can Exhibit Resistance To Stretching, Resulting In Pain And A Restricted Range Of Motion.

- Postural Instability Is A Common Symptom Of Parkinson's disease, Characterized By Difficulties In

Maintaining Balance And Coordination. This Can Significantly Raise The Likelihood Of Falling.

- Parkinson's disease can also Result in Additional Motor Symptoms, Including A Shuffling Gait, Reduced Arm Movement, And Challenges With Precise Motor Tasks.

Parkinson's disease Is Primarily Caused by the Gradual Deterioration of Neurons in the Substantia Nigra, A Region Of The Brain Responsible For Making Dopamine. Dopamine Is A Neurotransmitter That Has A Vital Function In Regulating Coordinated And Precise Motions. When Dopamine Levels Decline, The Motor Symptoms

Linked To Parkinson's disease Become Apparent.

The Precise Etiology Of The Degeneration Of Dopamine-Producing Neurons Remains Incompletely Elucidated, And Is Likely Multifactorial, Involving Both Hereditary And Environmental Influences. Several Possible Risk Factors Include Advanced Age, Genetic Susceptibility, Exposure To Specific Chemicals, And Other Unidentified Variables.

At Present, There Is No Known Remedy For Parkinson's Disease; Nonetheless, There Are Multiple Therapeutic Alternatives Accessible To Effectively Control Its Symptoms.

Levodopa And Other Medications Can Effectively Restore Dopamine Levels In The Brain. Physical Treatment, Occupational Therapy, And Lifestyle Adjustments Can Have A Substantial Impact On Enhancing The Quality Of Life For Those With Parkinson's disease.

Ongoing Research On Parkinson's Disease Is Progressing, And Improved Comprehension Of Its Mechanisms Holds The Potential To Pave The Way For Novel Treatment Strategies In The Future. Collaboration Between Persons With Parkinson's Disease And Healthcare Providers Is Crucial In Developing A Customized Treatment

Plan That Effectively Targets Their
Unique Requirements And Symptoms.

CHAPTER ONE
The Basics of Parkinson's Diet

Although There Is No Designated "Parkinson's Diet" That Will Cure Or Stop The Advancement Of Parkinson's Disease, Adhering To A Nutritious And Balanced Diet Can Significantly Contribute To Symptom Management And General Health. Below Are Some Overarching Dietary Recommendations That May Be Advantageous for Those Diagnosed with Parkinson's disease:

• Opt For A Diet That Is Well-Balanced And Incorporates A Diverse Range Of Foods That Are Rich In Nutrients. Incorporate Fruits, Vegetables, Whole Grains, Lean Meats, And Healthy Fats

Into Your Meals. This Can Aid In Delivering Vital Nutrients And Promoting Overall Well-Being.

• **Protein Management:** Certain Persons With Parkinson's Disease Observe That The Timing And Allocation Of Protein Consumption Throughout The Day Can Influence The Efficacy Of Their Medication, Specifically Levodopa. Engage In A Discussion With Your Healthcare Team To Ascertain The Optimal Protein Distribution For Your Prescription Regimen.

• Maintain Proper Hydration By Ensuring You Consume Enough Fluids. Dehydration Can Worsen Certain Symptoms Of Parkinson's Disease,

Such As Constipation. Ensuring Adequate Hydration Is Crucial For Maintaining Optimal Health.

• Incorporate Fiber-Rich Foods, Such As Whole Grains, Fruits, And Vegetables, Into Your Diet To Effectively Address Constipation, A Prevalent Problem Among Patients With Parkinson's Disease.

• Foods That Are Strong In Antioxidants Have The Potential To Safeguard Brain Cells From Harm. Incorporate Antioxidant-Rich Foods, Such As Berries, Leafy Greens, Nuts, And Seeds, Into Your Diet.

• Omega-3 Fatty Acids, Found In Fatty Fish (Salmon, Mackerel, And Trout),

Flaxseeds, And Walnuts, Have Anti-Inflammatory Characteristics And Can Be Advantageous For Brain Health.

• Sufficient Consumption Of Vitamin D Is Crucial For Maintaining Optimal Bone Health. To Obtain Natural Sunshine, It Is Advisable To Spend Time Outdoors. Additionally, It Is Recommended To Incorporate Vitamin D-Rich Foods Such As Fatty Fish, Fortified Dairy Products, And Eggs Into Your Diet.

• Reduce The Intake Of Processed Foods And Added Sugars: Limit The Consumption Of Food Products That Have Undergone Extensive Processing And Include High Amounts Of Added Sugars. Following A Diet That Is Low

In Added Sugars And Processed Foods Can Promote General Well-Being And Deter Weight Gain.

• **Personalized Approach:** Given The Varying Impact Of Parkinson's Disease On Individuals, It Is Essential To Customize Dietary Advice Based On Each Person's Own Requirements And Preferences. Seek Guidance From A Healthcare Practitioner Or A Qualified Dietitian To Develop A Customized Plan.

• **Medication And Diet Interaction:** Certain Drugs Prescribed For Parkinson's Disease May Have Interactions With Specific Foods Or Minerals. Ensure That You Engage In A Discussion With Your Healthcare

Practitioner Regarding Any Concerns Or Inquiries You May Have Concerning Potential Interactions.

Individuals With Parkinson's Disease Should Actively Cooperate With Their Healthcare Team, Which Includes A Certified Dietitian, To Create A Personalized Food Plan That Addresses Their Distinct Requirements And Effectively Manages Their Specific Symptoms. Periodic Surveillance And Modifications To The Dietary Regimen May Be Required Depending On Individual Reactions And Alterations In Health Condition.

Foods to Include

Including Nutrient-Rich Foods In Your Diet Can Support Overall Health And Potentially Help Manage Symptoms Associated With Parkinson's Disease. Here Are Some Foods To Consider Incorporating Into Your Diet:

- **Fruits And Vegetables:** These Are Rich In Vitamins, Minerals, Antioxidants, And Fiber. Aim for a Variety of Colorful Fruits and Vegetables to Ensure You're Getting a Wide Range of Nutrients. Berries, Leafy Greens, Broccoli, Carrots, Bell Peppers, And Citrus Fruits Are Particularly Nutritious Choices.

- **Whole Grains:** Whole Grains Provide Fiber, Vitamins, And Minerals.

Choose Whole Grains Such As Oats, Brown Rice, Quinoa, Barley, And Whole Wheat Bread Or Pasta Over Refined Grains.

• **Lean Proteins:** Protein Is Essential For Muscle Health And Overall Function. Opt For Lean Protein Sources Such As Poultry, Fish, Tofu, Beans, Lentils, And Low-Fat Dairy Products. Consider Distributing Your Protein Intake Evenly Throughout The Day To Avoid Interfering With The Absorption Of Levodopa.

• **Fatty Fish:** Fatty Fish Like Salmon, Mackerel, Sardines, And Trout Are Rich In Omega-3 Fatty Acids, Which May Have Anti-Inflammatory Properties And Support Brain Health.

• **Nuts And Seeds:** These Are Excellent Sources Of Healthy Fats, Protein, Vitamins, And Minerals. Incorporate Almonds, Walnuts, Flaxseeds, Chia Seeds, And Pumpkin Seeds Into Your Diet For Added Nutrients And Crunch.

• **Healthy Fats:** Include Sources Of Healthy Fats Such As Olive Oil, Avocado, And Fatty Fish To Support Heart And Brain Health.

• **Low-Fat Dairy:** Dairy Products Like Milk, Yogurt, And Cheese Provide Calcium, Vitamin D, And Protein. Opt For Low-Fat Or Non-Fat Varieties To Limit Saturated Fat Intake.

- **Legumes:** Beans, Lentils, Chickpeas, And Other Legumes Are Rich In Fiber, Protein, And Various Nutrients. They're Also Versatile and Can Be Included in Soups, Salads, Stews, and Side Dishes.

- **Herbs And Spices:** Incorporate Herbs And Spices Into Your Cooking To Add Flavor Without Extra Salt Or Unhealthy Fats. Turmeric, Ginger, Garlic, Cinnamon, And Rosemary Are Examples Of Flavorful Herbs And Spices With Potential Health Benefits.

- **Water:** Stay Hydrated By Drinking Plenty Of Water Throughout The Day. Proper Hydration Is Essential For Overall Health And Can Help Manage Symptoms Like Constipation.

Remember That Individual Dietary Needs May Vary, So It's Essential To Tailor Your Diet To Your Preferences, Health Goals, And Any Specific Dietary Restrictions Or Recommendations Provided By Your Healthcare Team. A Registered Dietitian Can Provide Personalized Guidance And Support In Creating A Balanced And Nutritious Diet Plan.

CHAPTER TWO
Foods to Limit or Avoid

Although There Is No Designated "Parkinson's Diet," Individuals With Parkinson's Disease Can Potentially Improve Symptom Management And General Health By Restricting Or Abstaining From Certain Foods. Here Are Some Factors To Take Into Account:

• **Excessive Protein:** Although Protein Is Necessary, Individuals With Parkinson's Disease May Experience Difficulties With The Absorption Of Levodopa, A Commonly Prescribed Medicine For Symptom Management, When Consuming A Diet High In Protein. It Is Advisable To Spread Out

Your Protein Consumption Throughout The Day And Consult Your Healthcare Practitioner To Determine The Best Timing For Optimal Results.

• Avoid Consuming Processed And Sugary Meals Due To Their Minimal Nutritional Content And Potential To Cause Weight Gain And Other Health Problems. Choose Entire, Nutrient-Rich Foods Instead.

• **High-Fat And Fried Foods:** Restrict The Consumption Of High-Fat And Fried Foods, Since They Might Potentially Lead To Weight Gain And May Not Be Beneficial For General Well-Being. Instead, Concentrate On Including Sources Of Nutritious Fats

Into Your Diet, Such As Avocados, Almonds, And Olive Oil.

• Elevated Sodium Consumption Might Potentially Exacerbate Hypertension, A Condition That May Be Of Particular Concern For Those Diagnosed With Parkinson's Disease. Restrict The Intake Of Processed And Packaged Foods That Contain Excessive Amounts Of Salt, And Opt For The Usage Of Herbs And Spices To Enhance The Taste Of Your Meals Instead.

• Alcohol Use In Large Amounts Can Have A Negative Impact On The Effectiveness Of Drugs And Worsen The Symptoms Of Parkinson's Disease. It Is Imperative To Engage In A Conversation With Your Healthcare

Practitioner Regarding Alcohol Usage And Contemplate Practicing Moderation Or Complete Abstinence.

• **Caffeine:** Although Consuming A Reasonable Amount Of Caffeine Is Generally Regarded As Harmless, Consuming An Excessive Amount Of Caffeine Can Disrupt Sleep And Contribute To Feelings Of Anxiety Or Restlessness. Due To Individual Variability In Tolerance, It Is Recommended To Closely Monitor The Effects Of Caffeine On Your Body And Make Necessary Adjustments.

• Avoid Taking Calcium Supplements In Close Proximity To Your Medicine, Since Calcium Can Hinder The Absorption Of Levodopa. In Addition,

Certain Foods That Are High In Iron, Such As Red Meat, Can Potentially Impact The Absorption Of Levodopa. Engage In A Conversation With Your Healthcare Physician Regarding Your Consumption Of Iron And Calcium In Your Diet.

• **Dairy Overconsumption:** Although Dairy Products Can Be Included In A Nutritious Diet, Individuals With Parkinson's Disease May Encounter Constipation, And Consuming An Excessive Amount Of Dairy Could Potentially Exacerbate This Problem. If You Are Experiencing Constipation, It Is Advisable To Consult Your Healthcare Professional To Explore Potential Dietary Modifications.

- **Constipation-Causing Foods:** People With Parkinson's Disease May Have A Higher Likelihood Of Experiencing Constipation. Restricting The Consumption Of Foods That Can Potentially Cause Constipation, Such As Processed Foods, Low-Fiber Foods, And Excessive Dairy Products, Can Be Advantageous.

- **Specific Stimuli:** Take Note Of How Particular Foods Impact Your Symptoms. Individuals With Parkinson's Disease May Have Symptom Triggers Or Worsening Of Symptoms After Consuming Specific Meals, Such As Spicy Dishes Or Those Containing High Levels Of Tyramine (Which Can Be Found In Old Cheeses,

Cured Meats, And Certain Fermented Foods). Identify And Restrict Any Specific Stimuli Based On Your Personal Encounters.

It Is Crucial To Seek The Assistance Of Healthcare Specialists, Such As A Certified Dietitian, While Making Dietary Modifications. This Will Ensure That Your Nutritional Plan Is Tailored To Your Own Health And Unique Requirements.

Meal Planning and Recipes

Meal Planning for Individuals with Parkinson's disease Involves Creating Balanced and Nutritious Meals That Address Specific Dietary Considerations and Support Overall Well-Being. Here Are Some Tips For Meal Planning And A Few Recipe Ideas:

Meal Planning Tips:

• **Balanced Meals:** Include A Variety Of Food Groups In Each Meal To Ensure A Balance Of Carbohydrates, Proteins, Healthy Fats, Vitamins, And Minerals.

• **Small, Frequent Meals:** Some People With Parkinson's Find It

Helpful To Have Smaller, More Frequent Meals Throughout The Day Rather Than Three Large Meals.

- **Protein Distribution:** If Taking Levodopa, Consider Distributing Protein Intake Evenly Throughout The Day To Avoid Interference With Medication Absorption.

- **Hydration:** Ensure Adequate Hydration By Drinking Water Throughout The Day. Dehydration Can Exacerbate Symptoms, Such As Constipation.

- **Fiber-Rich Foods:** Include High-Fiber Foods Like Whole Grains, Fruits, And Vegetables To Help Manage Constipation.

• **Easy-To-Chew Foods:** If Chewing Or Swallowing Is Challenging, Focus On Softer Foods Or Use Cooking Methods That Make Foods Easier To Chew.

• **Limit Processed Foods:** Minimize The Consumption Of Processed And Sugary Foods. Choose Whole, Nutrient-Dense Options Instead.

• **Adapt Recipes:** Modify Recipes To Meet Individual Preferences And Dietary Needs. Experiment With Herbs And Spices For Flavor Without Excessive Salt.

Sample Recipes:

1. Quinoa and Vegetable Stir-Fry:

Ingredients:

- 1 Cup Quinoa (Cooked)
- Mixed Vegetables (Broccoli, Bell Peppers, Carrots, Snap Peas)
- Tofu Or Chicken (Protein Source)
- Soy Sauce Or Tamari For Seasoning
- Garlic And Ginger For Flavor
- Sesame Oil For Cooking

Instructions:

- Stir-Fry Vegetables And Protein In Sesame Oil.
- Add Garlic And Ginger For Flavor.
- Mix In Cooked Quinoa And Soy Sauce/Tamari.

2. **Salmon and Avocado Salad:**

Ingredients:

- Grilled or Baked Salmon Fillet
- Mixed Salad Greens (Spinach, Arugula, Kale)
- Cherry Tomatoes, Cucumber, And Avocado
- Olive Oil And Lemon Juice For Dressing
- Optional: Nuts Or Seeds For Crunch

Instructions:

- Arrange Salad Greens On A Plate.
- Top With Grilled Salmon, Sliced Avocado, And Other Vegetables.

- Drizzle With Olive Oil And Lemon Juice.

3. **Sweet Potato and Lentil Soup:**

Ingredients:

- 1 Cup Red Lentils (Rinsed)
- 1 Large Sweet Potato (Peeled And Diced)
- Onion, Garlic, And Ginger For Flavor
- Vegetable Broth
- Turmeric And Cumin For Seasoning
- Coconut Milk (Optional)

Instructions:

- Sauté Onion, Garlic, And Ginger In A Pot.

- Add Lentils, Sweet Potato, Broth, And Spices.

- Simmer Until Lentils And Sweet Potatoes Are Cooked.

- Blend Part of the Soup For A Thicker Consistency.

4. Smoothie Bowl:

Ingredients:

- Frozen Berries (Blueberries, Strawberries)

- Banana

- Greek Yogurt Or Plant-Based Yogurt

- Spinach Or Kale (Optional)

- Toppings: Granola, Nuts, Seeds, Or Coconut Flakes

Instructions:

- Blend Berries, Banana, And Yogurt Until Smooth.
- Pour Into A Bowl And Add Desired Toppings.

Important Note:

Always Consult With A Healthcare Professional Or A Registered Dietitian For Personalized Advice Based On Individual Health Needs And Dietary Restrictions. They Can Provide Guidance On Specific Dietary Considerations Related To Parkinson's Disease And Help Create A Meal Plan That Aligns With Individual Health Goals.

CHAPTER THREE
Hydration and Parkinson's

Hydration Is Crucial For Overall Health, And It Is Particularly Important For Individuals With Parkinson's Disease. Proper Hydration Can Help Manage Symptoms, Support Medication Effectiveness, And Contribute To Overall Well-Being. Here Are Some Considerations And Tips For Staying Hydrated:

Importance of Hydration for Parkinson's:

• **Medication Absorption:** Some Medications Used To Manage Parkinson's Symptoms May Require Sufficient Water Intake For Optimal Absorption. It's Essential To Follow

Any Specific Recommendations Provided By Healthcare Professionals Regarding Medication And Hydration.

• **Constipation Management:** Parkinson's Disease Can Increase The Risk Of Constipation. Staying Hydrated Is Important For Maintaining Regular Bowel Movements And Preventing Constipation.

• **Temperature Regulation:** Parkinson's Can Affect The Body's Ability To Regulate Temperature. Proper Hydration Supports Temperature Regulation And Helps Prevent Issues Related To Overheating Or Dehydration.

- **Energy Levels:** Dehydration Can Contribute To Fatigue And Low Energy Levels. Staying Hydrated May Help Maintain Energy Throughout The Day.

Tips for Hydration:

- **Regular Water Intake:** Aim To Drink Water Consistently Throughout The Day. Carry A Water Bottle To Make It Easier To Track And Meet Your Hydration Goals.

- **Monitor Urine Color:** Check The Color Of Your Urine. Pale Yellow Or Light Straw Color Is Generally A Good Indication Of Adequate Hydration.

- **Flavor Water Naturally:** If Plain Water Is Unappealing, Add Natural

Flavor with Slices of Citrus Fruits, Cucumber, or Mint. Herbal Teas And Infused Water Can Also Be Refreshing Options.

- **Set Hydration Goals:** Establish Specific Hydration Goals Based On Your Individual Needs And Preferences. Work With Your Healthcare Team To Determine The Appropriate Amount Of Water For You.

- **Limit Caffeine And Alcohol:** Excessive Consumption Of Caffeine And Alcohol Can Contribute To Dehydration. If You Consume These Beverages, Balance Them With An Increased Intake Of Water.

- **Hydrating Foods:** Include Hydrating Foods In Your Diet, Such As Water-Rich Fruits And Vegetables (E.G., Watermelon, Cucumber, Celery).

- **Be Mindful Of Medication:** Some Medications May Increase The Risk Of Dehydration. Discuss With Your Healthcare Provider If You Are On Medications That May Impact Fluid Balance.

- **Address Swallowing Difficulties:** If Swallowing Is Challenging, Consider Consuming Hydrating Foods With Higher Water Content, Such As Soups, Smoothies, And Fruits.

Signs of Dehydration:

It's Important To Be Aware Of Signs Of Dehydration, Which Can Include Dark Urine, Dry Mouth, Increased Thirst, Fatigue, And Dizziness. If You Experience These Symptoms, Increase Your Fluid Intake And Consult With Your Healthcare Provider.

As Hydration Needs Can Vary Among Individuals, It's Crucial To Work Closely With Healthcare Professionals, Including A Registered Dietitian, To Develop A Personalized Hydration Plan That Meets Your Specific Needs And Helps Manage Symptoms Associated With Parkinson's Disease.

Overview of Common Supplements

While It's Important To Obtain Most Of Your Nutrients From A Well-Balanced Diet, Some People May Consider Supplements To Address Specific Nutritional Needs Or Deficiencies. Here's An Overview Of Some Common Supplements, Along With Their Potential Benefits And Considerations. Always Consult With A Healthcare Professional Before Starting Any New Supplement Regimen, As Individual Needs Can Vary:

Multivitamins:

• **Benefits:** Provides A Combination Of Essential Vitamins And Minerals To Support Overall Health.

- **Considerations:** Choose A Supplement With Appropriate Dosages, And Be Cautious Not To Exceed Recommended Levels, As Excessive Intake Of Certain Vitamins And Minerals Can Have Adverse Effects.

Vitamin D:

- **Benefits:** Supports Bone Health, Immune Function, And May Have A Role In Reducing Inflammation.

- **Considerations:** Adequate Sun Exposure, Fortified Foods, And Dietary Sources Like Fatty Fish Can Contribute To Vitamin D Intake. Discuss Supplementation With A Healthcare

Provider, Especially In Cases Of Deficiency.

Omega-3 Fatty Acids:

• **Benefits:** Supports Heart Health, Brain Function, And May Have Anti-Inflammatory Effects.

• **Considerations:** Sources Include Fatty Fish (Salmon, Mackerel), Flaxseeds, And Walnuts. Consider Supplementation If Dietary Intake Is Insufficient, But Consult With A Healthcare Provider For Guidance.

Calcium:

• **Benefits:** Essential For Bone Health And Muscle Function.

- **Considerations:** Dairy Products, Leafy Greens, And Fortified Foods Are Dietary Sources. Supplement If Dietary Intake Is Insufficient Or If There's A Medical Need. Avoid Exceeding Recommended Levels.

Iron:

- **Benefits:** Important For Oxygen Transport In The Blood And Overall Energy Levels.

- **Considerations:** Dietary Sources Include Red Meat, Beans, And Fortified Cereals. Iron Supplements May Be Recommended For Those With Deficiencies, But Excessive Intake Can Be Harmful.

B Vitamins (B6, B12, Folate):

- **Benefits:** Essential For Energy Metabolism, Nerve Function, And Red Blood Cell Formation.

- **Considerations:** Found In Various Foods, Including Meat, Poultry, Fish, And Leafy Greens. Supplements May Be Recommended For Certain Populations, Such As Vegetarians Or Those With Absorption Issues.

Magnesium:

- **Benefits:** Supports Muscle And Nerve Function, Bone Health, And Energy Production.

- **Considerations:** Dietary Sources Include Nuts, Seeds, Whole Grains, And Green Leafy Vegetables. Consult

With A Healthcare Provider Before Supplementing, As Excessive Magnesium Intake Can Have Adverse Effects.

Probiotics:

• **Benefits:** Supports Gut Health By Promoting The Growth Of Beneficial Bacteria.

• **Considerations:** Found In Fermented Foods (Yogurt, Kefir, Sauerkraut). Probiotic Supplements May Be Beneficial For Certain Digestive Issues, But Their Efficacy Can Vary.

Zinc:

- **Benefits:** Important For Immune Function, Wound Healing, And DNA Synthesis.

- **Considerations:** Dietary Sources Include Meat, Dairy, Nuts, And Seeds. Zinc Supplements May Be Recommended For Specific Populations Or Those With Deficiencies.

Coenzyme Q10 (Coq10):

- **Benefits:** Acts As An Antioxidant And Is Involved In Energy Production Within Cells.

- **Considerations:** Found In Small Amounts In Foods Like Fish, Meat, And Nuts. Coq10 Supplements May Be

Considered For Certain Conditions, But Consult With A Healthcare Provider.

Always Inform Your Healthcare Provider About Any Supplements You Are Taking, As They Can Interact With Medications Or Have Unintended Effects, Especially In High Doses. Individual Nutritional Needs Vary, And A Healthcare Professional Can Provide Personalized Advice Based On Your Health Status And Dietary Intake.

CHAPTER FOUR
Exercise and Its Impact on Parkinson's

Exercise Plays A Crucial Role In Managing The Symptoms Of Parkinson's Disease And Improving Overall Quality Of Life. Regular Physical Activity Has Been Shown To Have Several Positive Effects On Individuals With Parkinson's, Including Both Motor And Non-Motor Symptoms. Here Are Some Key Aspects Of How Exercise Impacts Parkinson's:

Motor Symptoms:

Improved Mobility and Balance:

• Exercise, Especially Activities That Focus On Balance And Coordination,

Can Enhance Mobility And Reduce The Risk Of Falls. Tai Chi, Yoga, And Specific Balance Exercises Can Be Beneficial.

Enhanced Strength and Flexibility:

• Resistance Training Helps Improve Muscle Strength, Flexibility, And Range Of Motion, Which Can Be Particularly Beneficial For Individuals With Parkinson's Who May Experience Stiffness.

Amelioration of Bradykinesia (Slowness Of Movement):

• Aerobic Exercises And Activities That Involve Repetitive, Rhythmic Movements, Such As Cycling, Walking,

Or Dancing, May Help Reduce Bradykinesia.

Tremor Management:

• While Exercise May Not Eliminate Tremors, It Can Help Improve Overall Muscle Control And Coordination, Potentially Reducing The Impact Of Tremors On Daily Activities.

Non-Motor Symptoms:

Improved Mood and Mental Well-Being:

• Exercise Has Been Shown To Boost Mood, Reduce Anxiety And Depression, And Improve Overall Mental Well-Being. This Is Particularly Important For Individuals With

Parkinson's, As They May Experience Mental Health Challenges.

Enhanced Cognitive Function:

• Physical Activity Has Cognitive Benefits And May Help Slow The Cognitive Decline Associated With Aging And Parkinson's Disease.

Better Sleep Quality:

• Regular Exercise Can Contribute To Better Sleep Quality, Which Is Often Disrupted In Individuals With Parkinson's.

Increased Energy Levels:

• Despite The Fatigue Often Associated With Parkinson's, Regular Exercise

Can Lead To Increased Energy Levels Over Time.

Neuroprotective Effects:

Potential Neuroplasticity:

• There Is Evidence To Suggest That Exercise May Promote Neuroplasticity, The Brain's Ability To Reorganize And Adapt, Potentially Providing A Protective Effect On The Brain's Structure And Function.

Release of Neurotrophic Factors:

• Exercise May Stimulate The Release Of Neurotrophic Factors, Which Are Proteins That Support The Growth, Survival, And Maintenance Of Neurons.

Recommendations for Exercise:

Aerobic Exercise:

• Activities Like Walking, Cycling, Swimming, And Dancing Can Improve Cardiovascular Fitness And Overall Well-Being.

Strength Training:

• Resistance Exercises Using Weights Or Resistance Bands Can Improve Muscle Strength And Flexibility.

Balance and Coordination Exercises:

• Tai Chi, Yoga, And Specific Balance Exercises Can Enhance Stability And Reduce The Risk Of Falls.

Flexibility Exercises:

• Stretching Exercises Can Help Improve Flexibility And Reduce Muscle Stiffness.

Individualized Approach:

• Exercise Programs Should Be Tailored To The Individual's Abilities, Preferences, And Specific Symptoms. Consultation With A Physical Therapist Or Exercise Professional Experienced In Working With Parkinson's Patients Is Beneficial.

Before Starting Any Exercise Program, Individuals With Parkinson's Should Consult Their Healthcare Provider, Particularly If They Have Specific Health Concerns Or Conditions That

May Impact Their Ability To Engage In Certain Activities. Additionally, Regular Reassessment And Adjustments To The Exercise Routine May Be Necessary Based On Individual Progress And Changing Health Status.

Preparing Parkinson's-Friendly Meals

When Preparing Meals For Individuals With Parkinson's Disease, It's Important To Consider Their Specific Needs, Such As Potential Swallowing Difficulties, Changes In Taste Perception, And Dietary Recommendations. Here Are Some Tips For Preparing Parkinson's-Friendly Meals:

1. **Texture Modifications:**

• Adjust Food Textures To Accommodate Any Swallowing Difficulties. This May Include Choosing Softer Foods, Using Sauces Or Gravies To Moisten Dishes, And Avoiding Overly Dry Or Tough Textures.

2. **Easy-To-Chew Foods:**

• Select Foods That Are Easy To Chew, Such As Cooked Vegetables, Tender Meats, And Ground Or Finely Chopped Options. Minimize Tough Cuts Of Meat And Offer Alternatives Like Poultry, Fish, Or Legumes.

3. **Finger Foods:**

• Consider Offering Finger Foods Or Bite-Sized Portions To Make It Easier

For Individuals With Fine Motor Skill Challenges To Handle Utensils.

4. **Flavor Enhancement:**

• Use Herbs, Spices, And Flavorful Ingredients To Enhance The Taste Of Meals. Parkinson's Disease Can Sometimes Affect Taste Perception, So Incorporating Bold Flavors Can Be Appealing.

5. **Hydration:**

• Include Hydrating Foods Like Soups, Stews, And Fruits To Support Overall Hydration, Especially If Swallowing Or Drinking Water Is Challenging.

6. **Balanced Nutrients:**

• Ensure Meals Are Well-Balanced With A Mix Of Protein, Carbohydrates, Healthy Fats, And A Variety Of Fruits And Vegetables.

7. **Individual Preferences:**

• Consider Personal Preferences And Dislikes. If Certain Foods Are More Appealing, Try To Incorporate Them Into The Diet To Encourage A Healthy Appetite.

8. **Consistent Meal Times:**

• Establish A Routine With Consistent Meal Times. This Can Help Regulate Medication Schedules And Create A Predictable Eating Routine.

9. **Assistive Devices:**

• Use Assistive Devices Such As Adapted Utensils Or Plate Guards If Needed To Make Eating More Manageable.

10. **Dysphagia Considerations:**

• If There Are Concerns About Swallowing Difficulties (Dysphagia), Consult With A Speech Therapist Or Healthcare Professional For Guidance On Appropriate Food Textures And Consistencies.

Sample Parkinson's-Friendly Recipes:

1. Soft Chicken And Vegetable Stew:

Ingredients:

- Tender Chicken Pieces
- Carrots, Potatoes, And Peas
- Low-Sodium Chicken Broth
- Herbs (Thyme, Rosemary)

Instructions:

1. Cook Chicken In A Slow Cooker With Vegetables And Herbs In Low-Sodium Broth Until Tender.
2. Serve The Stew In Bite-Sized Portions.

2. Salmon Salad with Avocado:

- Ingredients:
- Grilled Or Baked Salmon
- Mixed Greens
- Avocado Slices
- Cherry Tomatoes

- Olive Oil And Lemon Dressing
- Instructions:
- Arrange Mixed Greens On A Plate.
- Top With Grilled Salmon, Avocado, And Cherry Tomatoes.
- Drizzle With Olive Oil And Lemon Dressing.

3. **Soft Spinach And Cheese Omelette:**

Ingredients:

- Eggs
- Chopped Spinach
- Soft Cheese (Feta Or Goat Cheese)
- Herbs (Parsley, Chives)

Instructions:

- Whisk Eggs and Fold In Spinach And Cheese.
- Cook In A Non-Stick Pan Until Set.
- Sprinkle With Fresh Herbs Before Serving.

4. Smoothie Bowl:

Ingredients:

- Frozen Berries
- Banana
- Yogurt (Dairy Or Plant-Based)
- Toppings: Granola, Nuts, Seeds

Instructions:

- Blend Berries, Banana, And Yogurt Until Smooth.

- Pour into a Bowl and Top with Granola, Nuts, and Seeds.

Remember, Individual Preferences And Dietary Needs Can Vary, So It's Important To Tailor Meals To The Specific Tastes And Requirements Of The Person With Parkinson's Disease. Consult With Healthcare Professionals, Including A Dietitian Or Speech Therapist If Needed, To Ensure That The Meals Are Well-Suited To The Individual's Unique Needs And Challenges.

Conclusion

In Conclusion, Parkinson's Disease Presents Unique Challenges, But With Careful Management And Support, Individuals With Parkinson's Can Maintain A Good Quality Of Life. Understanding The Importance Of Factors Such As Exercise, Hydration, Medication Management, And Dietary Considerations Is Crucial For Effectively Managing Symptoms And Promoting Overall Well-Being.

• Regular Physical Activity, Including Aerobic Exercise, Strength Training, Balance, And Flexibility Exercises, Can Help Improve Mobility, Reduce The Risk Of Falls, Enhance Mood, And Support Cognitive Function.

Additionally, Staying Hydrated, Consuming A Balanced Diet Rich In Nutrients, And Considering Texture Modifications And Flavor Enhancements When Preparing Meals Can Make Eating More Enjoyable And Manageable For Individuals With Parkinson's.

• Collaboration With Healthcare Professionals, Including Neurologists, Physical Therapists, Occupational Therapists, Speech Therapists, Dietitians, And Other Specialists, Is Essential For Developing Personalized Treatment Plans And Addressing Individual Needs. Through A Holistic Approach That Considers Both Medical And Lifestyle Interventions,

Individuals With Parkinson's Disease Can Optimize Their Health And Quality Of Life.

While Parkinson's Disease Presents Challenges, It's Important To Focus On What Can Be Controlled And To Seek Support From Healthcare Providers, Family, And Community Resources. With Proper Management And Support, Individuals With Parkinson's Can Continue To Lead Fulfilling And Active Lives. Ongoing Research And Advancements In Treatment Offer Hope For Improved Outcomes And A Better Understanding Of The Disease In The Future.

THE END